Blood Pressure Measurement

Recommendations of the
British Hypertension Society

Blood Pressure Measurement

Recommendations of the British Hypertension Society

Third Edition

*These recommendations were prepared by the
Working Party on Blood Pressure Measurement
of the British Hypertension Society*

EOIN T O'BRIEN
*Blood Pressure Unit,
Beaumont Hospital, Dublin*

JAMES C PETRIE
University of Aberdeen

WILLIAM A LITTLER
University of Birmingham

MICHAEL DE SWIET
*Royal Postgraduate
Medical School, London*

PAUL L PADFIELD
University of Edinburgh

MICHAEL J DILLON
Hospital for Sick Children, London

ANDREW COATS
National Heart and Lung Institute, London

FÁINSIÁ MEE
*Nurses Hypertension Association,
Beaumont Hospital, Dublin*

BMJ Publishing Group

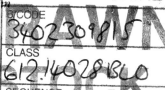

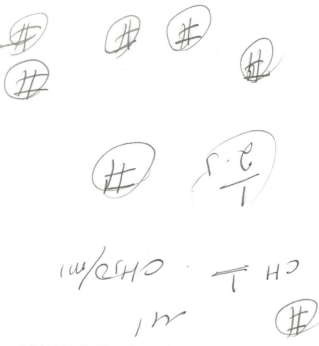

First Edition 1987
Reprinted 1988
Second Edition 1990
Reprinted 1991
Third Edition 1997

British Library Cataloguing in Publication Data
A catalogue record for this book is available from the British Library

ISBN 0–7279–1153–8

Typeset and printed in Great Britain by
Latimer Trend & Company Ltd, Plymouth

Introduction

Although conventional sphygmomanometry using the technique introduced by Riva-Rocci in 1896, and modified by Korotkoff in 1905, has served us well for the past hundred years, a new era has dawned. This third edition of the *Blood Pressure Measurement: Recommendations of the British Hypertension Society* differs, therefore, in emphasis from the first edition published in 1987.

Advances must be anticipated which herald new approaches to blood pressure measurement in practice. The development of reliable automated techniques of measurement has opened new possibilities, one example being the measurement of "ambulatory" blood pressure allowing recordings over 24 hours while subjects go about their daily activities.

The pressure from environmentalists to ban mercury as a toxic substance is likely to be persuasive, as indeed it has been in Scandinavian countries.

Although these developments may herald the demise of the conventional method of blood pressure measurement with the mercury sphygmomanometer, the technique is likely to remain in use for some time yet. The aim of these revised recommendations is to provide simple guidance for the indirect measurement of blood pressure while also anticipating how developments may influence practice.

Observer

Only an observer who is aware of the factors that lead to false readings should measure blood pressure. Inaccurate readings obtained through failure to use the proper technique lead to the wrong diagnosis, which may result in unnecessary or inappropriate treatment and follow up. Observer accuracy is often taken for granted but when doctors and nurses are assessed critically they may show a surprising degree of inaccuracy.

```
Incorrect technique→False readings
                  →Unnecessary treatment,
                   inappropriate treatment
                   and follow up
```

Procedure

Those who measure blood pressure should be familiar with the practical points listed and discussed below.

Practical points
- Explanation to patient
- White coat hypertension
- Defence reaction
- Variability in blood pressure
- Posture of patient
- Position of arm
- Application of cuff
- Position of manometer
- Estimation of systolic pressure
- Auscultatory measurement of systolic and diastolic pressure
- Number of measurements
- Indications for measurement in both arms
- Times of measurement
- Measurement in children
- Leaflet advice

Explanation to patient

The observer should outline the procedure briefly. In particular, he or she should warn the patient of the minor discomfort caused by inflation and deflation of the cuff and tell the patient that the measurement may be repeated several times.

White coat hypertension

In many patients blood pressure is always higher when measured by doctors (and nurses)—so called "white coat hypertension". Readings are likely to be lower when they are taken in the home or by ambulatory measurement.

Defence reaction

The defence reaction is the rise in blood pressure associated with the anxiety of measurement. This increase in blood pressure tends to subside once the patient becomes accustomed to the procedure and to the observer.

Changes in drug treatment should not be made on the basis of one measurement of blood pressure but rather on the patterns of blood pressure change during a period of observation. In many patients blood pressure levels fall without treatment.

Variability in blood pressure

Blood pressure varies in individuals according to the time of day, meals, smoking, anxiety, temperature, and the season of the year. It is usually at its lowest during sleep.

Posture of patient

Whether the patient is sitting or lying (supine) makes no difference to the blood pressure readings. However, pressure should also be measured in the standing position in patients whose symptoms or drug regimen may be associated with a disproportionate postural fall. Pregnant patients may suffer a profound fall in blood pressure when lying supine; therefore in pregnancy all measurements should be performed with the patient either sitting or in the left lateral position. No information is available on the optimal time to be spent in a particular position before the measurement. We suggest three minutes lying or sitting and one minute standing.

Position of arm

The arm should be horizontal and supported at the level of the mid-sternum because dependency of the arm below heart level leads to an overestimation of systolic and diastolic pressures of about 10 mm Hg. Correspondingly, raising the arm above the heart level leads to underestimation of these pressures.

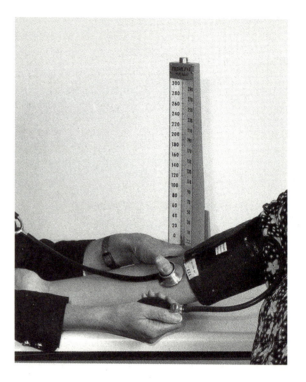

Application of cuff

The patient should be in a warm environment. Tight or restrictive clothing should be removed from the arm. A simple measure is to request that patients wear a short sleeved garment when attending for blood pressure measurement.

The position of maximal pulsation of the brachial artery in the arm, just above the antecubital fossa, may be marked lightly with a pen. A cuff with a long enough bladder should then be applied to the upper arm. Since contact of the stethoscope with the tubing of the cuff may produce artefactual sounds, the tubing from the blood pressure cuff should not cross the auscultatory area. The centre of the bladder should be positioned over the line of the artery. The lower edge of the bladder should be 2–3 cm above the marked point. The cuff should fit firmly and comfortably and be well secured.

Position of manometer

In the mercury column manometer the column must be vertical (unless designed with a tilt), at eye level, and not more than three feet from the observer. Stand mounted manometers are recommended, largely because they are mobile and easily adjusted for height. Box and desk models are more easily damaged and less convenient to use.

Estimation of systolic pressure

The systolic pressure should be estimated before the operator uses the stethoscope by palpating the brachial artery pulse and inflating the cuff until the pulsation disappears. The point of disappearance represents the systolic pressure. This measure is especially useful in patients in whom auscultatory end points may be difficult to judge accurately—for example, pregnant women, patients in shock, or those taking exercise.

Auscultatory measurement of systolic and diastolic pressures

The stethoscope is placed gently over the artery at the point of maximal pulsation. It must not be pressed too firmly or touch the cuff, or the diastolic pressure may be underestimated. The pressure is then raised by inflating the bladder to 30 mm Hg above the systolic blood pressure as estimated by palpation. Next the pressure is reduced at 2–3 mm Hg per second. The point at which repetitive, clear tapping sounds first appear for at least two consecutive beats gives the *systolic blood pressure*. The point where the repetitive sounds finally disappear gives the *diastolic blood pressure* (phase 5). Both measurements should be taken to the nearest 2 mm Hg.

Auscultatory sounds

- *Phase 1* The first appearance of faint, repetitive, clear tapping sounds which gradually increase in intensity for at least two consecutive beats is the systolic blood pressure
- *Phase 2* A brief period may follow during which the sounds soften and acquire a swishing quality
- *Auscultatory gap* In some patients sounds may disappear altogether for a short time
- *Phase 3* The return of sharper sounds, which become crisper to regain, or even exceed the intensity of phase 1 sounds. The clinical significance, if any, to phases 2 and 3 has not been established
- *Phase 4* The distinct abrupt muffling sounds, which become soft and blowing in quality
- *Phase 5* The point at which all sounds finally disappear completely is the diastolic pressure

Palpatory estimation of systolic pressure

(1) Palpate brachial artery pulsation
(2) Inflate cuff until pulsation vanishes
(3) Deflate cuff
(4) Estimate systolic pressure

Auscultatory measurement of systolic and diastolic pressure

(5) Place stethoscope gently over point of maximal pulsation of brachial artery
(6) Inflate cuff to 30 mm Hg above estimated systolic pressure
(7) Reduce pressure at rate of 2–3 mm Hg per second or per pulse beat
(8) Take reading of systolic pressure when repetitive, clear tapping sounds appear for two consecutive beats
(9) Take reading of diastolic pressure when repetitive sounds disappear

Digit preference, whereby observers choose to record a favourite number, most commonly 0 or 5 mm Hg, is a serious source of bias. It is important to realise that such digit preference may introduce substantial errors that could lead to incorrect decisions being made, especially in patients with borderline blood pressures. Such bias is best avoided by recording systolic and diastolic pressures to the nearest 2 mm Hg.

The *silent or auscultatory gap* occurs when the sounds disappear between the systolic and diastolic pressures. The importance of the gap is that unless the systolic pressure is palpated first it may be underestimated. The presence of a silent gap should be recorded on the case sheet or blood pressure chart.

Number of measurements

It is preferable to take one measurement carefully at each visit, repeating the measurement if there is uncertainty or distraction, rather than making a number of hurried measurements. If the blood pressure is elevated above say 140/90 mm Hg, a second reading should be recorded after an interval of at least one minute. For patients in whom sustained increases of blood pressures are being assessed a number of measurements should be made on different occasions before definite diagnostic or management decisions are made.

Sustained blood pressure elevation

Repeat measurement at least once at each visit on the same arm

Make a number of measurements at different visits

Make each measurement carefully

Indications for measurement in both arms

The pulse should always be palpated in both arms. A difference between arm pulses may be a clue to coarctation of the aorta, anatomical variants and alterations to the pulse following surgical or cardiological procedures, such as cardiac catheterisation.

Blood pressure should be measured in both arms in all patients with raised blood pressure at the initial assessment. It is suggested that if there is a reproducible difference of 20 mm Hg for systolic pressure and 10 mm Hg for diastolic pressure decision making should be based on the limb with the higher pressure. Simultaneous measurement in both arms is indicated in patients with suspected coarctation of the aorta where local anatomical abnormalities are suspected.

What to note when measuring blood pressure
- The blood pressure should be written down as soon as it has been recorded
- Measurements of systolic and diastolic pressure should be made to the nearest 2 mm Hg
- Pressures should not be rounded off to the nearest 5 or 10 mm Hg—digit preference
- The arm in which the pressure is being recorded and the position of the subject should be noted e.g. left arm, sitting
- Pressures should be recorded in both arms on first attendance
- In obese patients the arm circumference and bladder size should be indicated
- In clinical practice the diastolic pressure should be recorded as phase 5 except in those patients in whom sounds persist greatly below muffling; this should be clearly indicated e.g. 154/68/10
- If the patient is anxious, restless or distressed, a note should be made with the blood pressure
- The presence of an auscultatory gap should always be indicated e.g. 166/94 (A.G from 158–142)

Coarctation of aorta or suspected anatomical abnormalities

Measure simultaneously in both arms

Times of measurement for patients taking drugs that lower blood pressure

In patients taking drugs that lower blood pressure the measurements may vary depending on the time of day at which the drugs are taken. It may therefore be helpful, when assessing the effect of antihypertensive drugs, to note the time of drug ingestion in relation to the time of measurement.

Obtaining a blood pressure profile

Accurate though measurement may be when the above recommendations are followed, it should be realised that any such measurement represents only a fraction of the 24-hour blood pressure profile. The increasing use of 24-hour ambulatory blood pressure measurement in clinical practice has shown a number of patterns of blood pressure behaviour, such as the "white coat" effect whereby the circumstances of measurement may in themselves induce a rise in blood pressure. It is, therefore, important to attempt to obtain a profile of blood pressure behaviour. This may be best achieved by 24-hour ambulatory measurement, but repeated measurements of blood pressure at successive visits home recording also give helpful information on blood pressure behaviour.

For the future, careful measurement of blood pressure with a mercury sphygmomanometer following the above recommendations is likely to remain the most effective first line in assessing blood pressure. If conventional measurement is below 150/90 mm Hg, especially over a number of measurements, that individual may be passed as normotensive. If, however, blood pressure is elevated above this level an assessment of blood pressure behaviour should be obtained before diagnostic and therapeutic decisions are made.

Self (home) measurement

Blood pressure measured in the home is usually lower than that recorded by a doctor or nurse in a clinical setting. Home measurement of blood pressure has failed to achieve the success and popularity of home blood sugars in diabetic patients, mainly because of the inaccuracy of blood pressure measuring devices. The advent of accurate and inexpensive automated devices which can provide a print-out of blood pressure measurement with time and date should remove many of the drawbacks and lead to increased attention to home blood pressure measurement.

Ambulatory blood pressure measurement (ABPM)

The increased demand for 24-hour blood pressure measurement has resulted in the production of a variety of ambulatory devices. Ambulatory systems must be accurate, reasonably priced and the recorders should be compact, noiseless, and light and comfortable for the patient to wear. In obese patients a cuff containing an appropriately sized bladder must be used.

● The operator must:
be familiar with the equipment
know the calibration procedures for the device
know the normal ranges of blood pressure during the day and night

---

Suggested diagnostic thresholds for 24-hour ambulatory pressure rounded for ease of use in clinical practice

	Normotensive levels	Definitely hypertensive levels
Daytime pressure	<135/85	≥ 140/90
Night-time pressure	<120/70	≥ 125/75

The relationship of these levels to clinical outcome awaits the results of ongoing research.

---

be aware of the factors influencing the diurnal pattern
give the necessary time to instruct the subject so as to obtain as many measurements as possible during the recording period

- Subjects for ABPM must be capable of coping with and caring for the recorder
- Normal activity should be maintained during ABPM except when measurements are being made by the recorder
- Subject's arm should be still during measurement
- Similar levels of activity for comparative repeat measurements
- Working days should not be compared with recreational days
- Comparative measurements in shift workers should be made between similar shifts
- For clinical use recordings are usually programmed for every 30 minutes
- Subjects should keep a diary of activities and symptoms during the recording period

The clinical indications for ABPM are growing. The following constitute the main uses:

- Borderline hypertension
- White coat hypertension
- Isolated systolic hypertension in the elderly
- Assessment of nocturnal blood pressure
- Resistant hypertension
- Evaluation of hypotensive symptoms
- Miscellaneous diagnostic uses

"White coat hypertension"

This may be defined simply as a rise in blood pressure associated with the procedure of having blood pressure measured. It may result partly from anxiety but in many subjects there is a deeper "learning" process which may condition the rise in blood pressure for the procedure of measurement. Whatever the mechanism, the reality is that as many as 10–20% of patients labelled as having "hypertension" using conventional blood pressure measurement may have "white coat hypertension" and may not require blood pressure lowering drugs. ABPM is the most effective method of determining whether blood pressure elevation is the result of "white coat hypertension".

"White coat effect"

This may be defined as a rise in blood pressure in patients with hypertension associated with the procedure of having blood pressure measured. It occurs in many hypertensive patients and its clinical importance is that patients with hypertension may appear more hypertensive than is the case if ABPM is used to assess blood pressure elevation.

Equipment

Mercury sphygmomanometers

The mercury sphygmomanometer was introduced to clinical medicine by Scipione Riva-Rocci in 1896. A decade later Nikolai Korotkoff discovered that sounds are audible as an occluding cuff was deflated and the stethoscope became as indispensable to the measurement of blood pressure as the mercury manometer. It is likely that this traditional technique which has contributed so much to our knowledge of hypertension over the past century will soon disappear from clinical practice. There are three reasons for this eventuality: mercury is likely to be banned from hospital use because of the danger of toxicity, accurate automated devices are now available to replace the mercury sphygmomanometer and with the advent of 24 hour ambulatory blood pressure measurement into clinical practice, more reliance is being placed on blood pressure behaviour than on casual measurement of blood pressure levels.

Banning mercury from the wards raises another issue of even greater importance for clinical medicine than that of rendering the mercury sphygmomanometer obsolete. If the millimetre of mercury is no longer the unit of measurement for blood pressure, there can be little scientific argument against its replacement with the *Système International* (SI) unit, the kilopascal.

The British Hypertension Society has instructed its Working Party on Blood Pressure Measurement to consider the implications of these issues for clinical practice and to draw up recommendations for the smooth implementation of the necessary changes required. Towards this end the equivalent value of the kilopascal against the millimetre of mercury is shown in the table.

Table of equivalence of units

mm Hg	kPa
1	0·1
2	0·2
3	0·4
4	0·6
5	0·7
6	0·8
7	0·9
8	1·0
9	1·2
10	1·4
20	2·6
30	4·0
40	5·4
50	6·7
60	8·0
70	9·4
80	10·7
90	12·0
100	13·4
110	14·7
120	16·0
130	17·4
140	18·7
150	20·0
160	21·4
170	22·7
180	24·0
190	25·4
200	26·7
250	33·4
260	34·7
270	36·0
280	37·4
290	38·7
300	40·0

Shaded areas = decision pressures
1 mm Hg = 0·133 kPa exactly
1 kPa ≃ 8 mm Hg

kPa rounded to nearest decimal point
Current scale markings of 2 mm Hg ≃ 0·25 kPa

The mercury sphygmomanometer consists of a manometer, an inflatable bladder in a cuff, and an inflation–deflation device. Before any measurement is attempted the equipment must be checked to make sure that it is appropriate and in good order. If any part of the apparatus is defective or unsuitable, alternative equipment must be used.

Points to check in assessing equipment
Manometer—visibility of meniscus; calibration
Cuff—condition; length and width of inflatable bladder
Inflation–deflation device—possible malfunction; control valve
Stethoscope—condition
Maintenance—regularity; responsibility

Features affecting accuracy of the mercury sphygmomanometer
- When the sphygmomanometer is not in use, the top of the mercury meniscus should rest at exactly zero without pressure applied; if it is below this the device needs to be serviced.
- The scale should be clearly calibrated in 2 mm divisions from 0 to 300 mm Hg and should indicate accurately the differences between the levels of mercury in the tube and in the reservoir
- The diameter of the reservoir must be at least 10 times that of the vertical tube, or the vertical scale must correct for the drop in the mercury level in the reservoir as the column rises
- Substantial errors may occur if the manometer is not kept vertical during measurement. Calibrations on floor models are especially adjusted to compensate for the tilt in the face of the gauge. Stand mounted manometers are recommended for hospital use. This allows the observer to adjust the level of the sphygmomanometer and to perform measurement without having to balance the sphygmomanometer precariously on the side of the bed
- The air vent at the top of the manometer must be kept patent as clogging will cause the mercury column to respond sluggishly to pressure changes and to overestimate pressure
- The control valve is one of the commonest sources of error in sphygmomanometers and when it becomes defective it should be replaced. Spare control valves should be available in hospitals and a spare control valve should be supplied with sphygmomanometers

Advice to be included in the instructions accompanying a sphygmomanometer using mercury

Guidelines and precautions

A mercury-type sphygmomanometer should be handled with care. In particular, the instrument should not be dropped or treated in any way that could result in damage to the manometer. Regular checks should be made to ensure that there are no leaks from the inflation system and that the manometer has not been damaged so as to cause a loss of mercury.

Health and safety when handling mercury

Exposure to mercury can have serious toxicological effects; absorption of mercury results in neuropsychiatric disorders and, in extreme cases, nephrosis. Therefore precautions should be taken when carrying out any maintenance to a mercury sphygmomanometer.

All maintenance necessitating handling of mercury should be conducted by the manufacturer or specialised service units.

Mercury spillage

When dealing with a mercury spillage, wear latex gloves. Avoid prolonged inhalation of mercury vapour. Do not use an open vacuum system to aid collection.

Collect all the small droplets of split mercury into one globule and immediately transfer all the mercury into a container, which should then be sealed.

After removal of as much of the mercury as practicable, treat the contaminated surfaces with a wash composed of equal parts of calcium hydroxide and powdered sulphur mixed with water to form a thin paste. Apply this paste to all the contaminated surfaces and allow to dry. After 24 hours, remove the paste and wash the surfaces with clean water. Allow to dry and ventilate the area.

Manometer

Mercury column manometer The meniscus should be clearly visible and not be obscured by oxidised mercury on the inside of the glass. Before inflation it must be at zero.

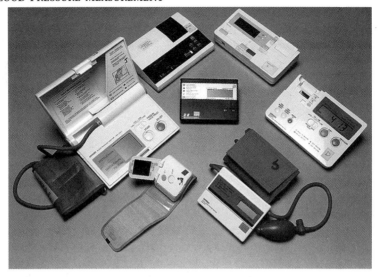

Automated devices for measuring blood pressure in the home; some of these may be suitable for measuring blood pressure in the clinical setting.

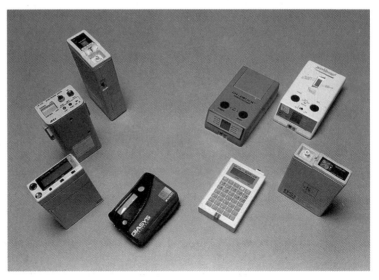

Automated devices for measuring ambulatory blood pressure.

Aneroid sphygmomanometers

Aneroid sphygmomanometers were once popular because they were more compact than mercury sphygmomanometers, but their use is now discouraged because their accuracy deteriorates with use, leading usually to falsely low readings and a consequent underestimation of blood pressure. If an aneroid sphygmomanometer is used, its accuracy may be checked at different pressure levels by connecting it with a Y piece to the tubing of a standardised mercury column manometer. If recalibration is necessary this must be done by the manufacturer.

Automated devices

Most automated devices work on one of three principles—the detection of Korotkoff sounds by a microphone or the detection of arterial blood flow by ultrasound or oscillometry. Until recently automated devices depended on Korotkoff sound detection using an electronic microphone shielded from extraneous noise in the pressure cuff with blood pressure being recorded on a print-out or indicated on a digital display. The microphones are sensitive to movement and friction, however, and may be difficult to place accurately. Manufacturers are turning, therefore, to oscillometric detection of blood pressure in which cuff placement is not critical. Until recently the accuracy of automated devices was questionable but accurate automated sphygmomanometers for clinic or home measurement are now available, though tests of reliability after a period of time in use have not been performed. As with all equipment, the user is advised to seek independent evidence of validation from the manufacturer.

Cuff

The cuff consists of an inflatable bladder within a restrictive cloth sheath. The bladder, tubing, connections, inflation bulb, and valves should all be sound. The sheath containing the bladder should also be in good condition and have a secure fastening. Provided it is long enough to wrap round the arm and be easily secured, the length of the sheath is not important.

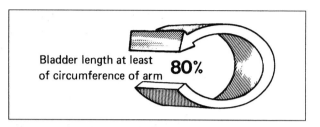

Bladder length at least **80**% of circumference of arm

Bladder dimensions

Miscuffing

Too narrow or too short a bladder will cause overestimation of blood pressure. Too wide or too long a bladder may cause underestimation of blood pressure. The former has the effect in clinical practice of overdiagnosing and the latter of underdiagnosing hypertension. Either error has serious implications.

Provided bladder length is such as to encircle 80% of arm circumference, bladder width is not so critical provided it is not less than 12 cm. Most arms do not readily accommodate bladders with widths greater than 13 cm as the bladder is likely to encroach on the antecubital fossa.

● Bladder too small = *undercuffing* = overestimation of BP
● Bladder too large = *overcuffing* = underestimation of BP
  undercuffing more common than *overcuffing*

Arm circumference

The mean arm circumference in many European countries averages about 30 cm. Knowing that measurement will be most accurate with a cuff containing a bladder that will encircle 80% of arm circumference it can be calculated that a bladder measuring 12 × 26 cm would correctly cuff 79% of European arms, incorrectly cuff 21% of arms, 10% from undercuffing and 11% from overcuffing. Further a bladder that is suitable for Northern Europeans may be too large for the leaner arms of, for example, Brazilians.

These findings suggest that the optimum bladder dimensions should be recommended according to the arm circumference of the population for which the recommendation applies. It would seem appropriate, therefore, to have available three cuffs containing bladders with the following dimensions:

- A standard bladder measuring 12×26 cm for the majority of adult arms
- An "obese" bladder measuring 12×40 cm for obese arms
- A "small" bladder measuring 10×18 cm for lean adult arms and children

Footnote: *In its previous recommendations, the British Hypertension Society Working Party recommended a cuff containing a bladder 12×35 cm on the basis that such a cuff would give accurate blood pressure measurements in the majority of adults.*

The dimensions of the bladder should be clearly shown on each cuff, together with a prominent marker indicating the centre of the bladder.

Recommended bladder dimensions

Dimensions	Subject	Maximum arm circumference
4×13 cm	Small children	17 cm
10×18 cm	Medium sized children and lean adults	26 cm
12×26 cm	Majority of adult arms	33 cm
12×40 cm	Obese adults	50 cm

Accurate readings may be obtained in adults with arm circumferences greater than 50 cm by placing a cuff with a 40 cm bladder so that the centre of the bladder is over the brachial artery. All dimensions to have a tolerance of ±1 cm.

Inflation–deflation device

Failure to achieve a pressure of 40 mm Hg above the estimated systolic blood pressure or 200 mm Hg after 3–5 seconds of rapid inflation is a sign of possible equipment malfunction. So too is the inability of the equipment to deflate smoothly when the controlling release valve is operated at 2–3 mm/s or at each pulse beat. When such problems occur the unit should be set aside and clearly marked with instructions for defective parts to be repaired or replaced. Faulty control valves, leaks, dirty vents, and perished tubing are simple to repair. The commonest source of error in the inflation–deflation system is the control release valve, which can easily be replaced.

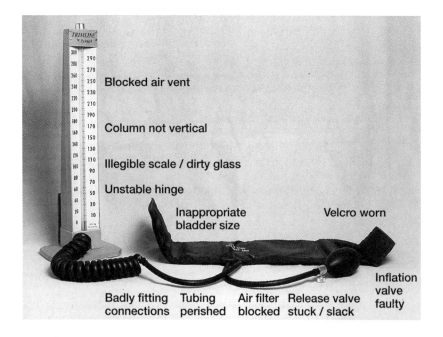

Deflation that is either jerky or too rapid may result in the systolic pressure being underestimated and the diastolic pressure overestimated. If, on the other hand, deflation is too slow the patient may suffer pain, even bruising, and blood pressure may be overestimated.

Stethoscope

The stethoscope should be a good quality one in good condition with clean, well fitting earpieces.

Maintenance

The due date of next servicing should be clearly marked on the sphygmomanometer. Sphygmomanometers should be serviced every six months. Replacement parts are cheap and should be readily available in the clinical area, together with a maintenance instruction booklet.

The responsibility for reporting faulty equipment or the lack of appropriate cuffs lies with the observer, who should always refuse to use defective or inappropriate equipment. The responsibility for arranging regular maintenance should be clearly defined for each clinical area.

Sphygmomanometer maintenance

Responsibility for maintenance clearly defined
Date for routine 6-monthly service marked on unit
Defective equipment reported to member of staff responsible
Replacement parts and instruction booklet available in clinical
area

Leaflet advice

Patients with high blood pressure should be given a leaflet stressing that blood pressure elevation is only one risk factor for cardiovascular disease. Giving up cigarettes, reducing alcohol consumption, weight reduction, and dietary restrictions of cholesterol and fats, may be as important as lowering blood pressure.

21

The following should be your goals

1. If you smoke—stop now
2. Your ideal body weight is ....
3. To achieve this your total daily calorie intake should not exceed ....
4. If your diet is high in cholesterol—reduce your consumption of cholesterol rich foods
5. Do not add salt to food at table
6. Take regular exercise
7. If tablets are prescribed take these as instructed and never stop tablets without consulting your doctor

The successful management of blood pressure depends on cooperation between the patient and the doctor.

What is blood pressure?

Everyone has a certain level of blood pressure. It is the force of the blood from the heart against the walls of the arteries.

About one in five adults develop high blood pressure for reasons that are not fully understood, and this is often called hypertension.

High blood pressure means that the heart has extra work to do and it increases in size to overcome the pressure. Also the blood vessels thicken to contain the higher pressure of the blood. This reaction in the heart and blood vessels leads to heart disease, and vascular disease such as stroke.

What is normal blood pressure?

Blood pressure is measured with a sphygmomanometer which gives two pressure levels in millimetres of mercury—written as mm Hg; the high level is the systolic pressure and the low level is the diastolic pressure. Blood pressure varies considerably with activity, emotion, stress, age and a number of other factors, but in adults persistent elevation of pressure above 150/90 (Systolic/Diastolic) mm Hg is an indication for medical advice.

Blood pressure measurement in special circumstances

Children

The only technique that is at present practical for widespread clinical application is conventional sphygmomanometry using a well-maintained mercury sphygmomanometer. Systolic blood pressure is preferred to diastolic blood pressure because of its greater accuracy and consistency.

The choice of the correct cuff is crucial. To cover the age range from 0–14 years a minimum of three cuffs is necessary with the bladder dimensions—4×13 cm, 10×18 cm, and 12×26 cm (adult size). The widest cuff that can be applied to the arm should be used. The length of the bladder should be such as to encircle 80% of the arm circumference. Secure fastening is essential and may not be possible with velcro especially when using the small cuffs.

In some healthy children aged under 5 years and all children under 1 year, measurement of blood pressure by conventional sphygmomanometry is impossible because the Korotkoff sounds cannot be heard reliably. In these and children who are shocked or have low cardiac outputs, more sensitive detection systems, such as Doppler ultrasound or oscillometry, should be used. *Circumstances of measurement* Except in acutely ill children, blood pressure should be measured after the child has been sitting quietly (or lying if aged under 2) for at least three minutes. Measurements made when the child is eating, sucking, or crying will be unrepresentative and usually too high. Management decisions should not be taken on the basis of specialist advice. In older children the indications for ambulatory blood pressure measurement are the same as for adults.

Obesity

In obese subjects the arm circumference is increased. The "standard" cuff may lead to blood pressure being erroneously elevated—so called "cuff hypertension". All physicians should have a large cuff (bladder dimensions 12×40 cm) available as obesity is quite commonly associated with raised blood pressure. Failure to take arm circumference into account may have serious implications for the management of patients.

Arrhythmias

The major source of difficulty in blood pressure measurement in arrhythmias is that when cardiac rhythm is irregular there is a large variation in blood pressure from beat to beat. Thus in arrhythmias, such as atrial fibrillation, stroke volume and as a consequence blood pressure, vary depending on the preceding pulse interval. Blood pressure measurement in atrial fibrillation, particularly when the ventricular rhythm is highly irregular, will at best constitute a rough estimate, the validity of which can perhaps be improved upon only by using repeated measurements.

Pregnancy

Between 2% and 5% of pregnancies in Western Europe are complicated by clinically relevant hypertension. In a significant number of these raised blood pressure is a key factor in medical decision-making in the pregnancy. Particular attention must be paid to blood pressure management in pregnancy because of the important implications for patient management as well as the fact that it presents some special problems.

Recent studies have resolved the controversy as to whether the muffling or disappearance of sounds should be taken for diastolic blood pressure. Disappearance of sounds (fifth phase) is now recommended for the measurement of diastolic pressure.

Elderly people

The combination of hypertension and ageing is manifest as a decrease in arterial compliance. There is also deterioration in baroreceptor and autonomic function. The consequences are a variety of blood pressure manifestations in elderly hypertensives; which include the following:

● Isolated systolic hypertension
● Increased variability of blood pressure
● "White coat" isolated systolic hypertension
● Postural hypotension
● Post-prandial hypotension
● Autonomic failure resulting in low day-time/high night-time BP

Conclusions

● The measurement of blood pressure is one of the most commonly performed procedures in clinical medicine and should be done carefully.

● The main cause of misleading readings should be highlighted in training.

● All those who measure blood pressure should be assessed on the practical aspects of the procedure.

● Defective or inappropriate equipment must not be used. A phased maintenance programme is essential and inexpensive.

● A maintenance programme should be defined for each clinical area where blood pressure measurements are made.

● Mercury is a toxic substance. Care must be exercised when handling mercury sphygmomanometers and special precautions taken if mercury spillage occurs.

● Automated devices will in time replace mercury sphygmomanometers. Such devices must be subjected to independent validation of accuracy.

● Special consideration has to be given to the technique of blood pressure measurement in special groups, such as children, the obese, the elderly, and pregnant women.

Index